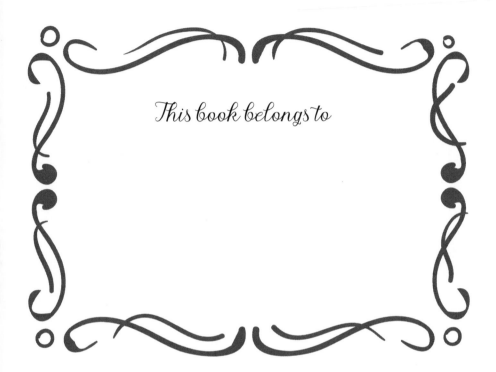

This book belongs to

Game Rules

for couple

Take turns and choose between
TRUTH or **DARE**.

If you don't answer the truth question or complete
your dare, your partner can choose your "punishment".

P.s. You are only allowed 5 truths!

Game Rules

for party with "friends"

Every player sits in a circle, then an empty bottle is placed on a table or on the ground.

- Palyer 1 begins by rotating the bottle.

  The bottleneck now points to player 2.

- Player 2 choose **TRUTH** or **DARE**

  If a dare is chosen, player 2 turns the bottle again to find his/her dare partner!

If player 2 does not answer the truth question or complete his/her dare, player 1 can choose his/her "punishment"!

P.s. Each player are only allowed 5 truths!

#1
TRUTH

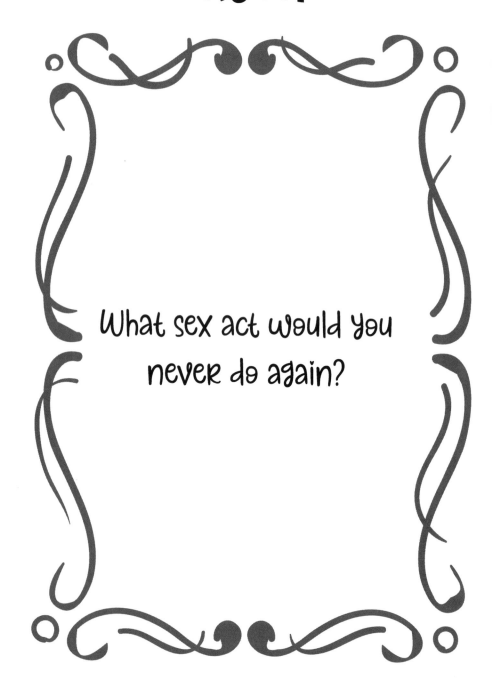

What sex act would you
never do again?

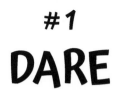

#1
DARE

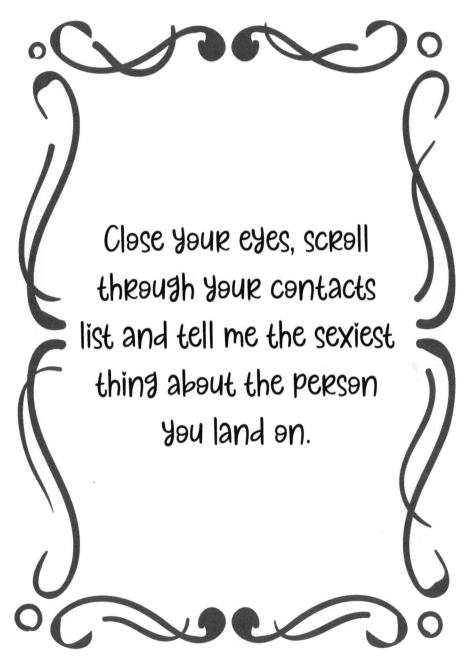

Close your eyes, scroll
through your contacts
list and tell me the sexiest
thing about the person
you land on.

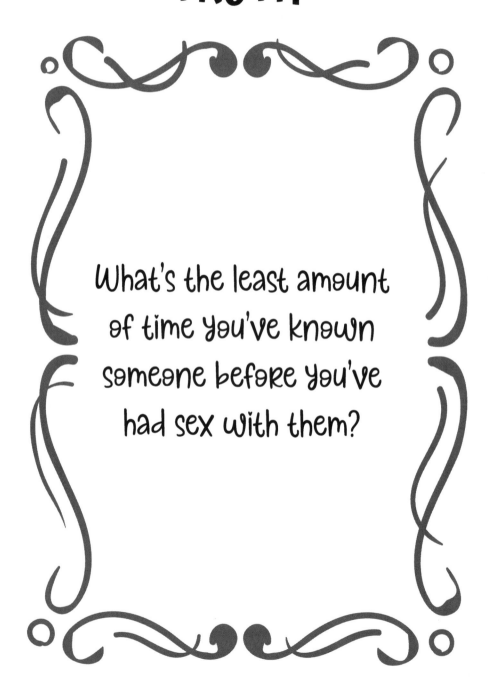

#2
TRUTH

What's the least amount
of time you've known
someone before you've
had sex with them?

#2
DARE

Sing the chorus of a song
you've had sex to.

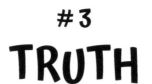

#3
TRUTH

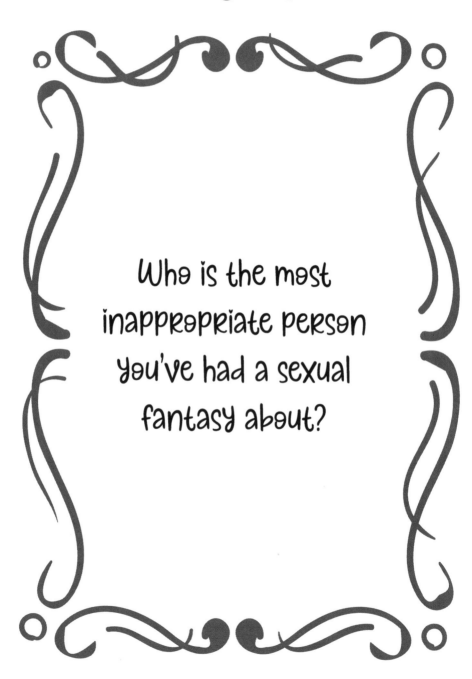

Who is the most
inappropriate person
you've had a sexual
fantasy about?

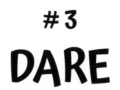

#3
DARE

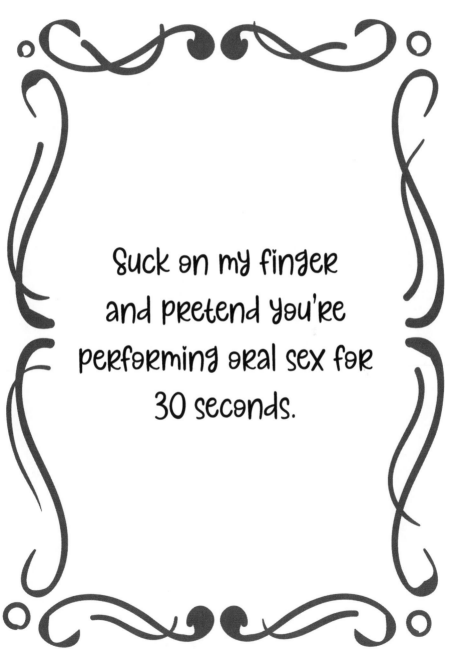

Suck on my finger
and pretend you're
performing oral sex for
30 seconds.

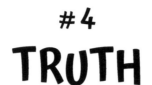

#4
TRUTH

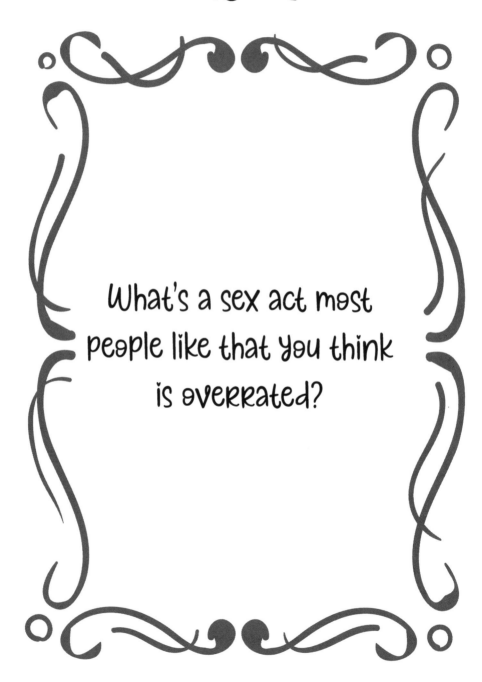

What's a sex act most
people like that you think
is overrated?

#4
DARE

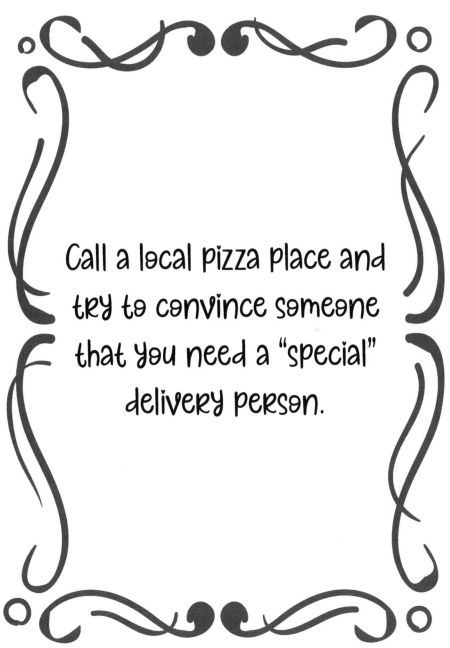

Call a local pizza place and try to convince someone that you need a "special" delivery person.

#5
TRUTH

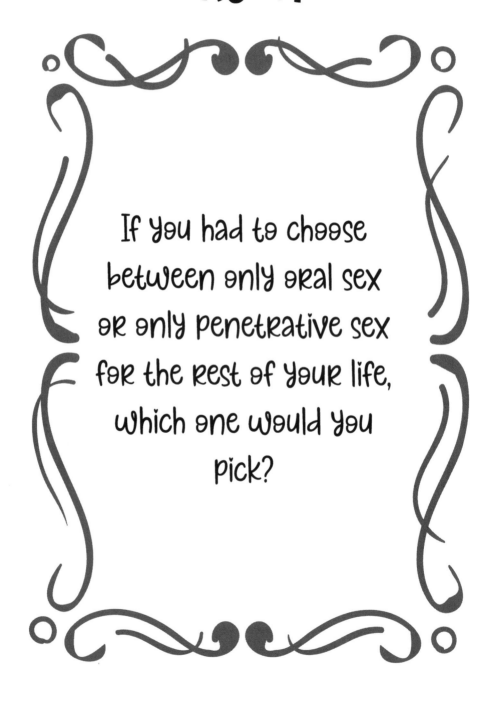

If you had to choose between only oral sex or only penetrative sex for the rest of your life, which one would you pick?

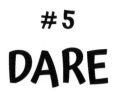

#5
DARE

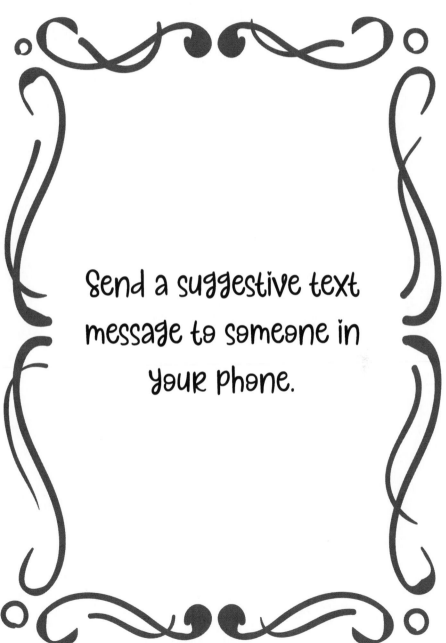

Send a suggestive text
message to someone in
your phone.

TRUTH

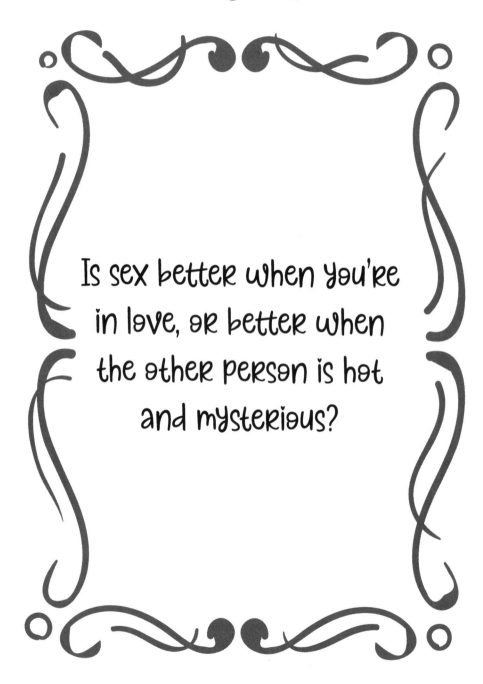

Is sex better when you're in love, or better when the other person is hot and mysterious?

DARE

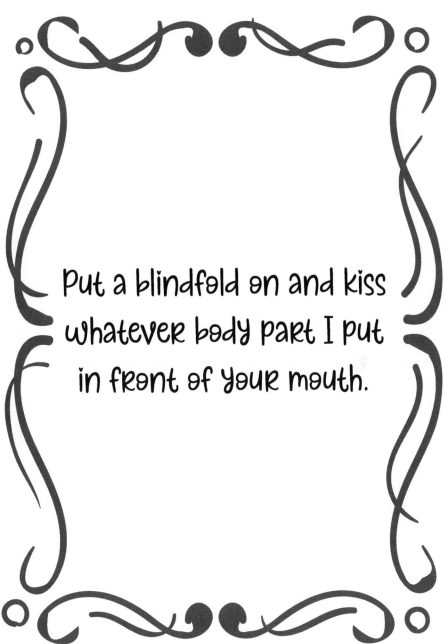

Put a blindfold on and kiss
whatever body part I put
in front of your mouth.

TRUTH

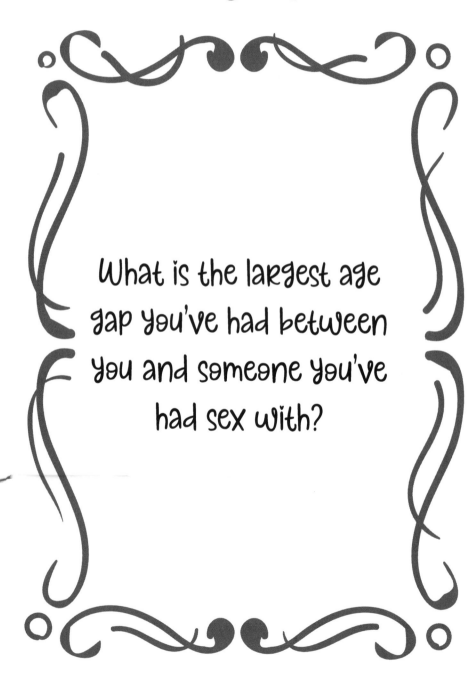

What is the largest age
gap you've had between
you and someone you've
had sex with?

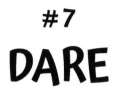

#7
DARE

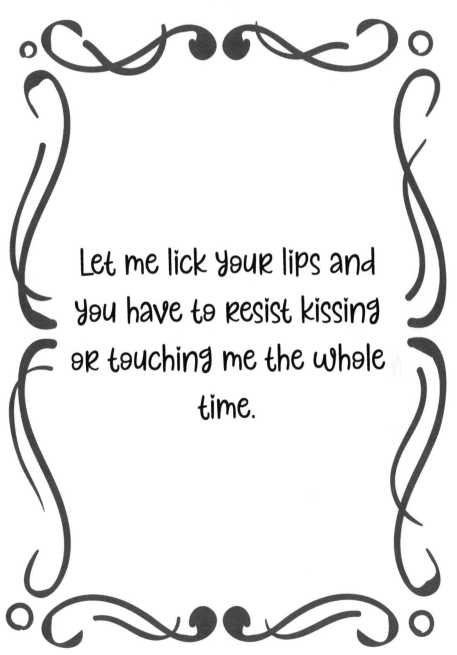

Let me lick your lips and you have to resist kissing or touching me the whole time.

TRUTH

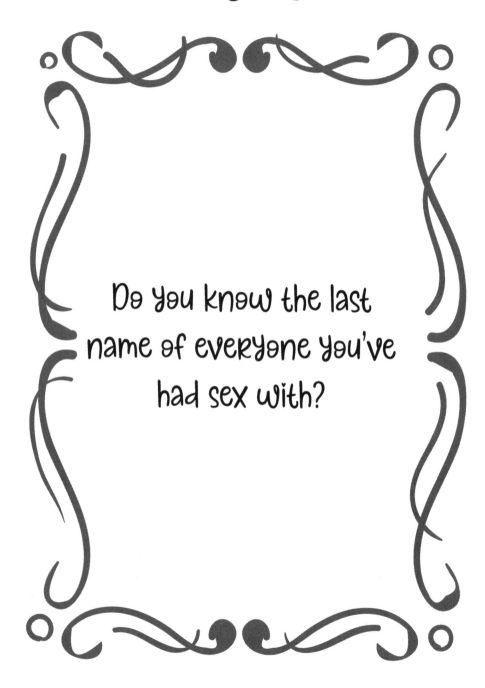

Do you know the last name of everyone you've had sex with?

#8
DARE

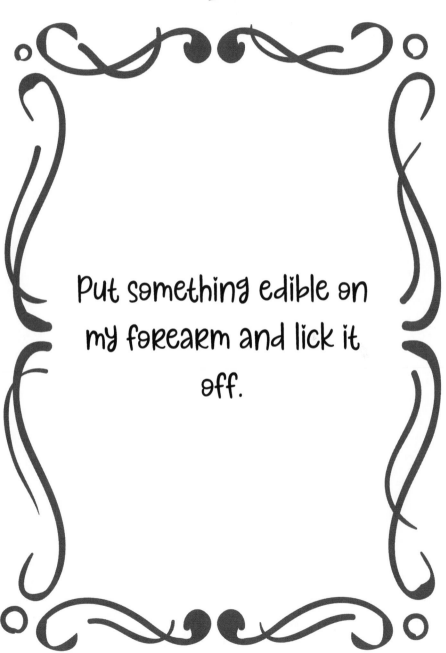

Put something edible on
my forearm and lick it
off.

TRUTH

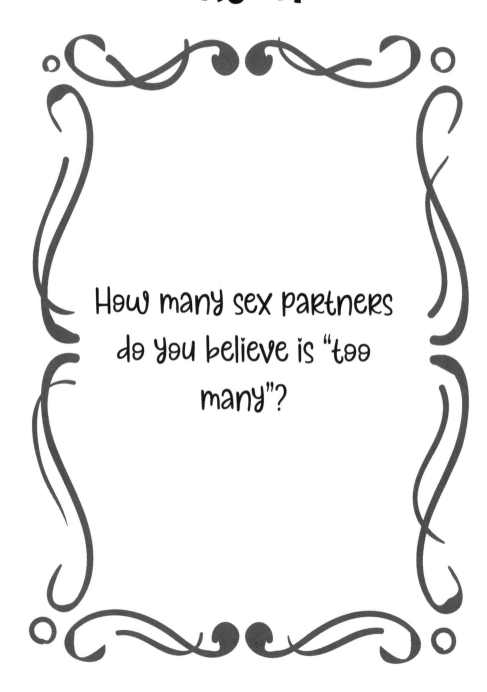

How many sex partners do you believe is "too many"?

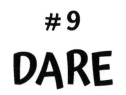

#9
DARE

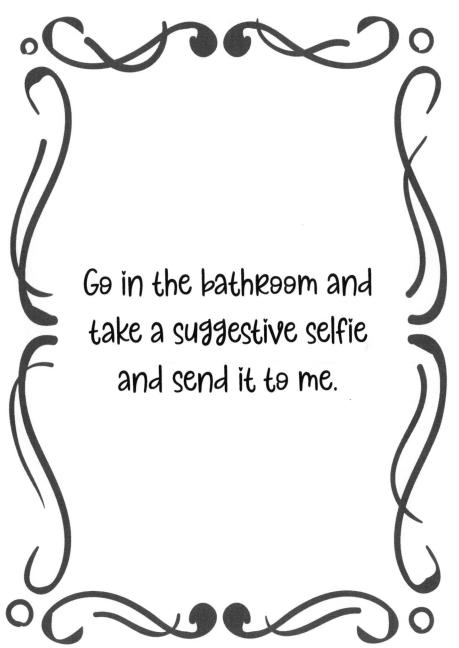

Go in the bathroom and
take a suggestive selfie
and send it to me.

#10
TRUTH

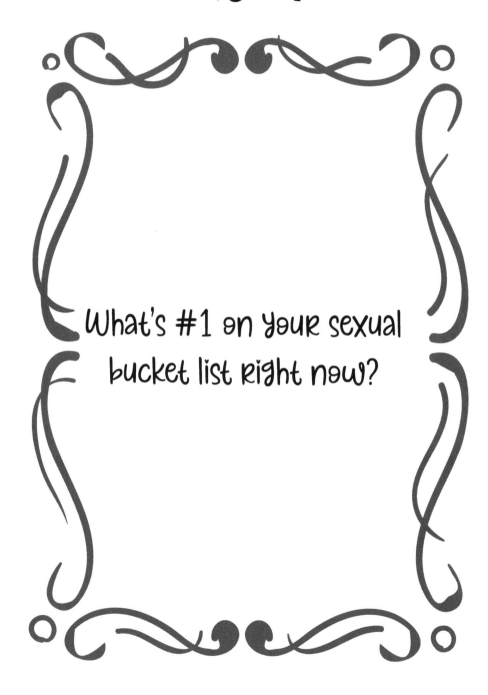

What's #1 on your sexual bucket list right now?

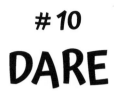

#10
DARE

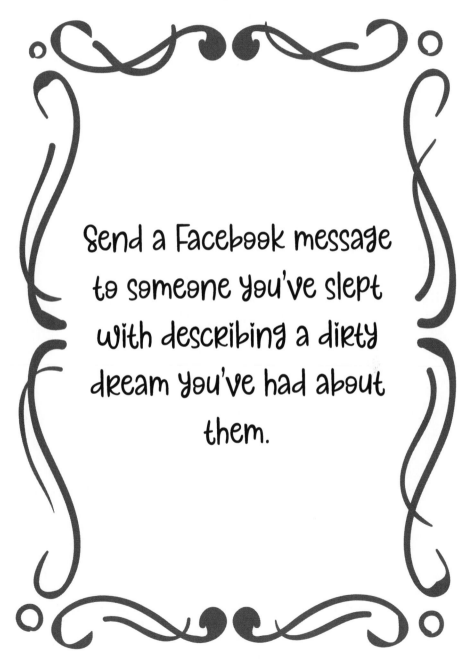

Send a Facebook message to someone you've slept with describing a dirty dream you've had about them.

#11
TRUTH

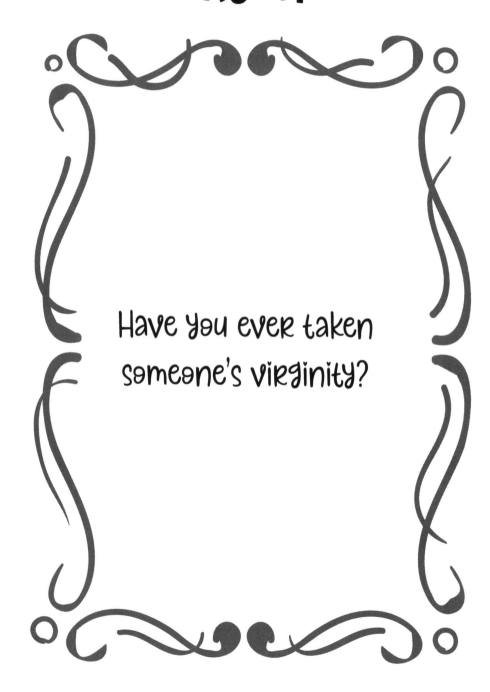

Have you ever taken
someone's virginity?

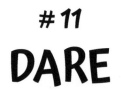

#11
DARE

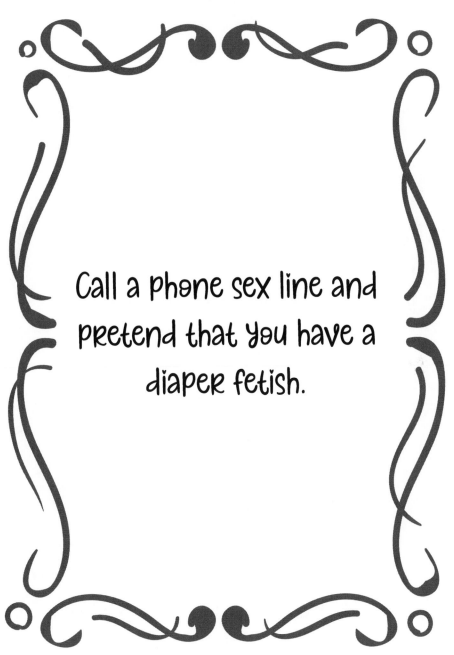

Call a phone sex line and pretend that you have a diaper fetish.

12
TRUTH

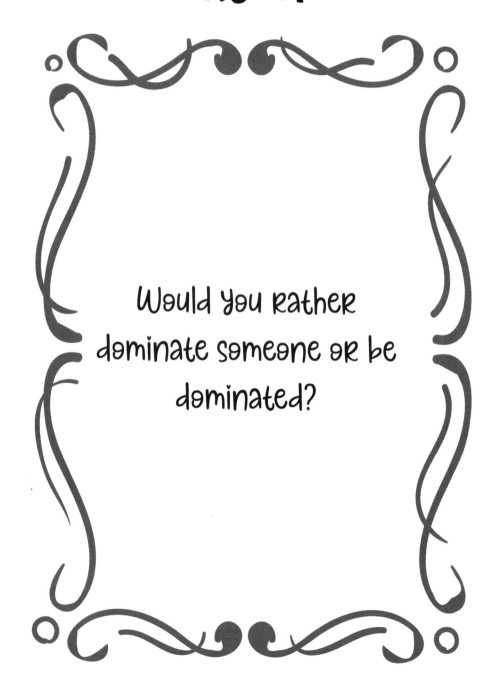

Would you rather dominate someone or be dominated?

DARE

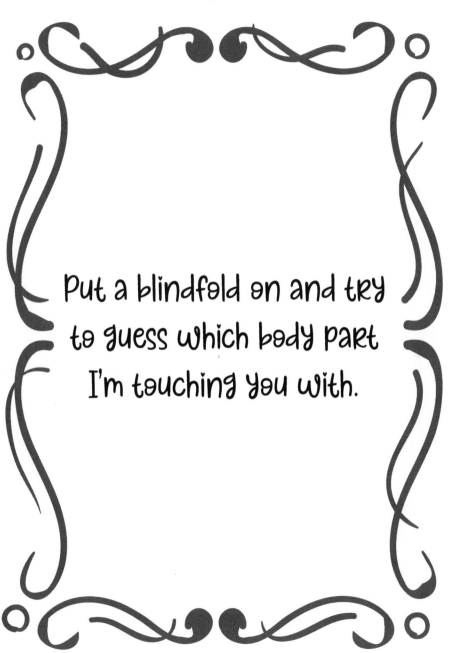

Put a blindfold on and try
to guess which body part
I'm touching you with.

#13
TRUTH

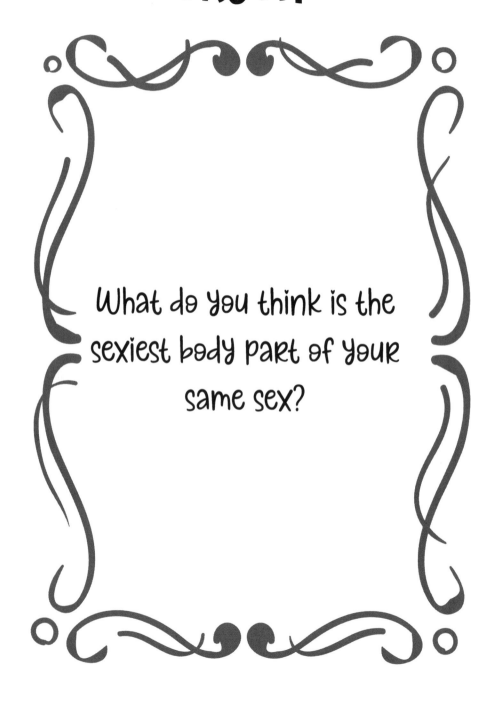

What do you think is the
sexiest body part of your
same sex?

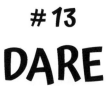

#13
DARE

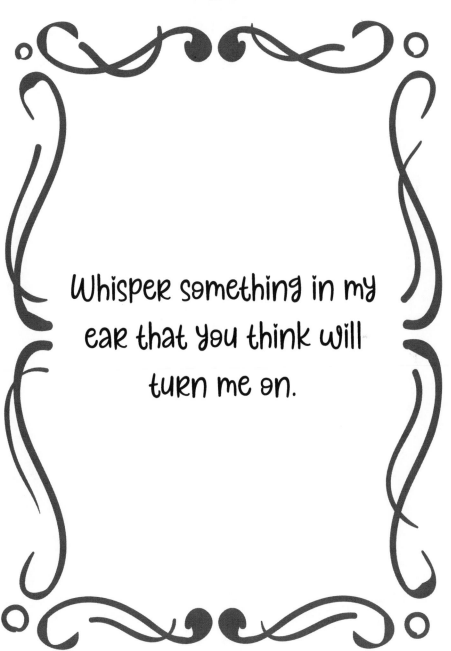

Whisper something in my ear that you think will turn me on.

#14
TRUTH

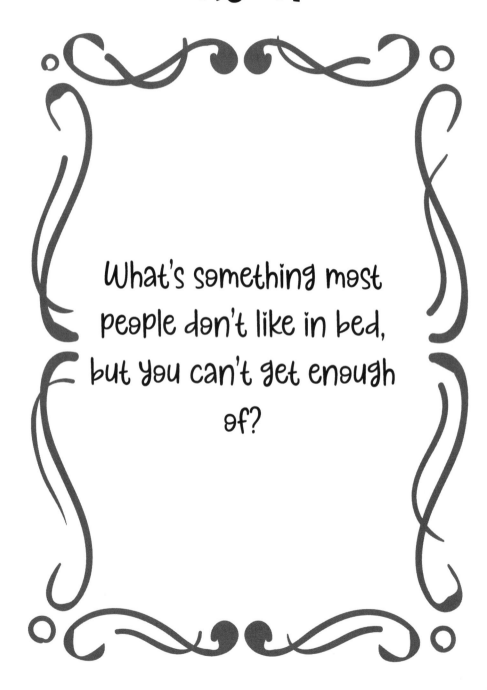

What's something most people don't like in bed, but you can't get enough of?

DARE

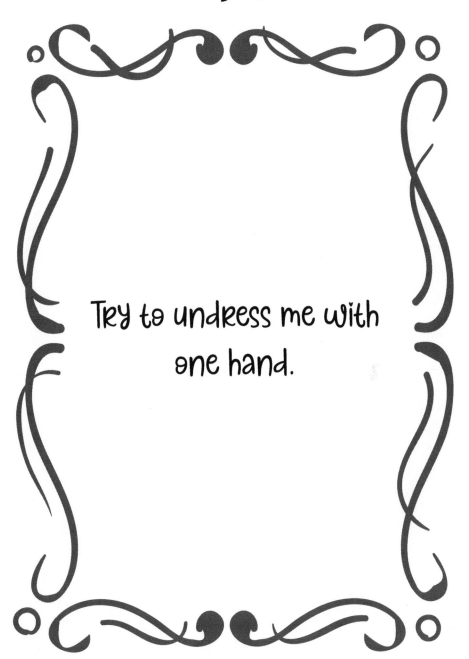

Try to undress me with one hand.

#15
TRUTH

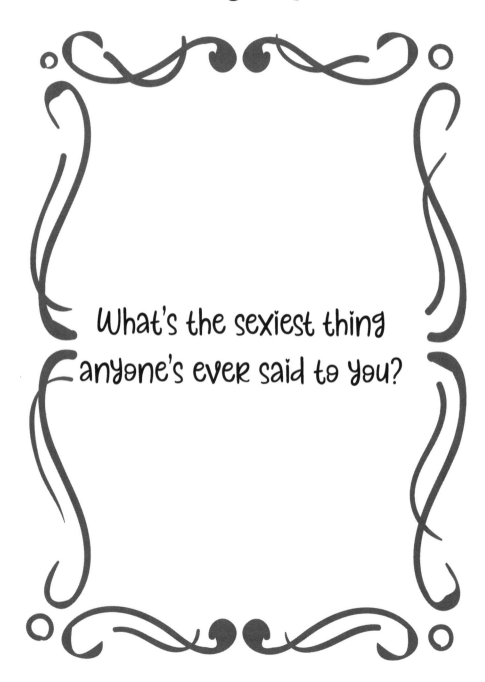

What's the sexiest thing
anyone's ever said to you?

#15
DARE

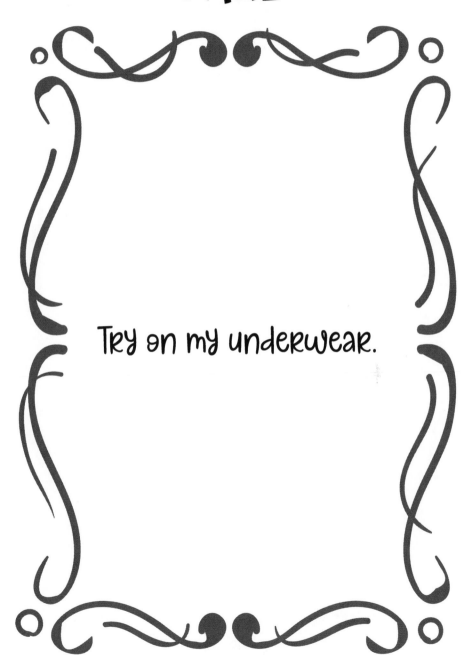

Try on my underwear.

TRUTH

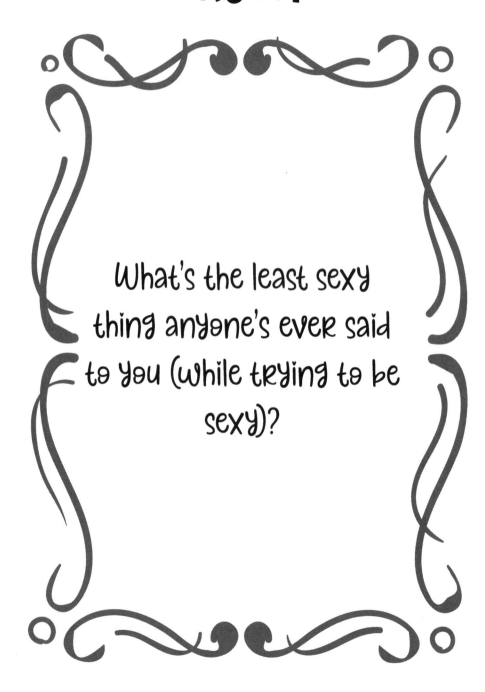

What's the least sexy thing anyone's ever said to you (while trying to be sexy)?

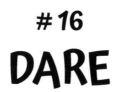

#16
DARE

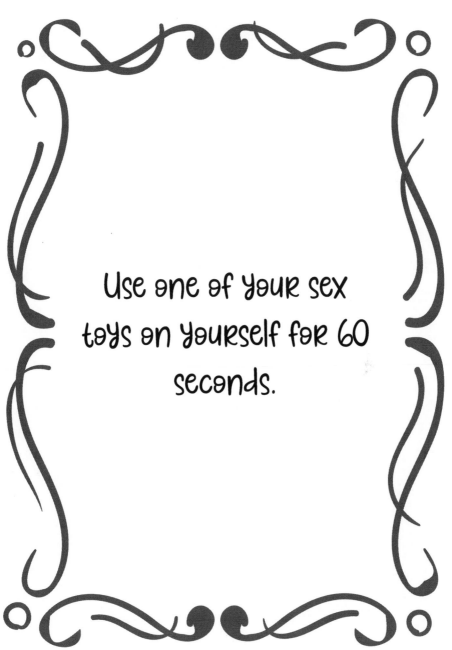

Use one of your sex toys on yourself for 60 seconds.

TRUTH

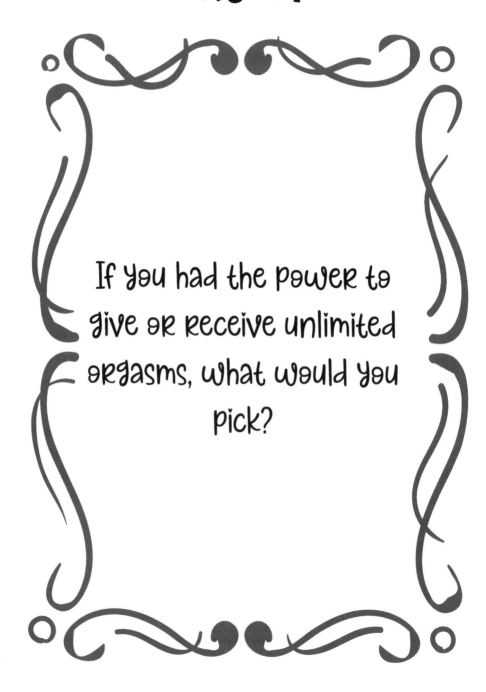

If you had the power to give or receive unlimited orgasms, what would you pick?

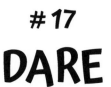

17
DARE

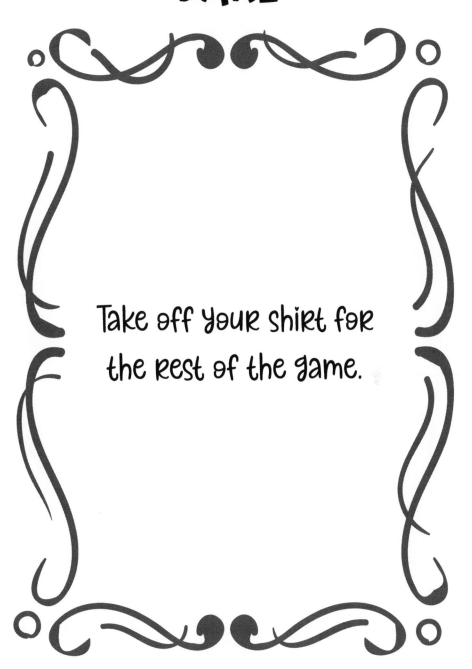

Take off your shirt for
the rest of the game.

#18
TRUTH

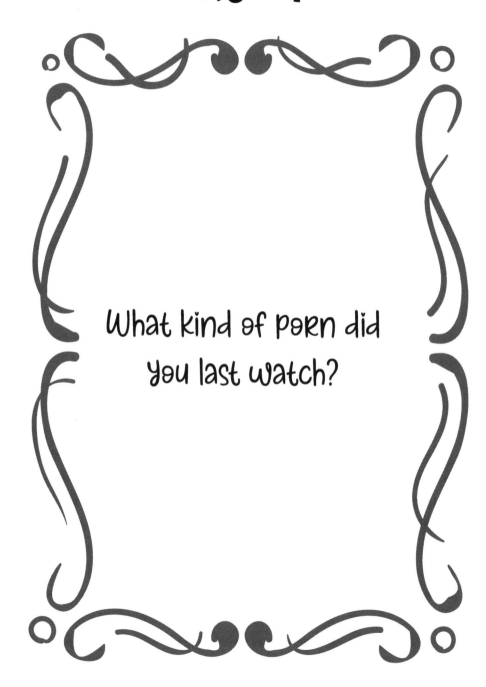

What kind of porn did
you last watch?

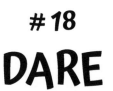

#18
DARE

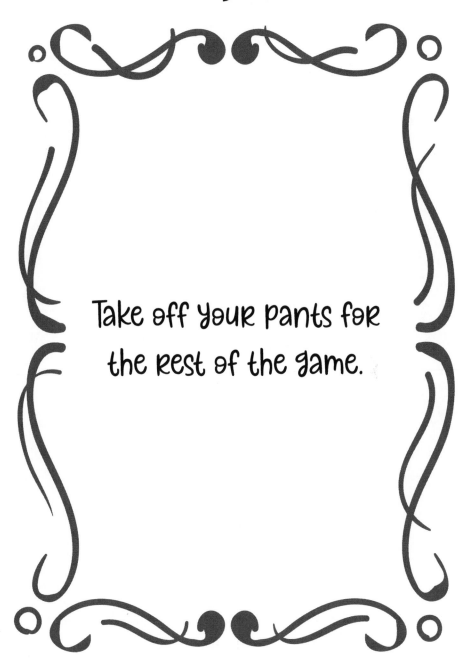

Take off your pants for
the rest of the game.

TRUTH

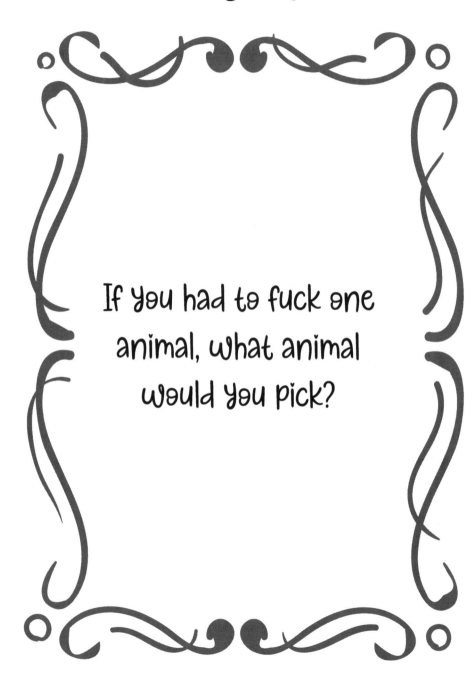

If you had to fuck one
animal, what animal
would you pick?

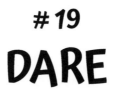

#19
DARE

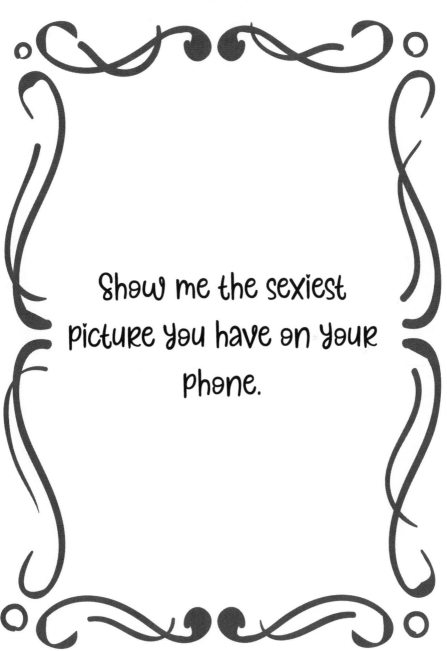

Show me the sexiest picture you have on your phone.

TRUTH

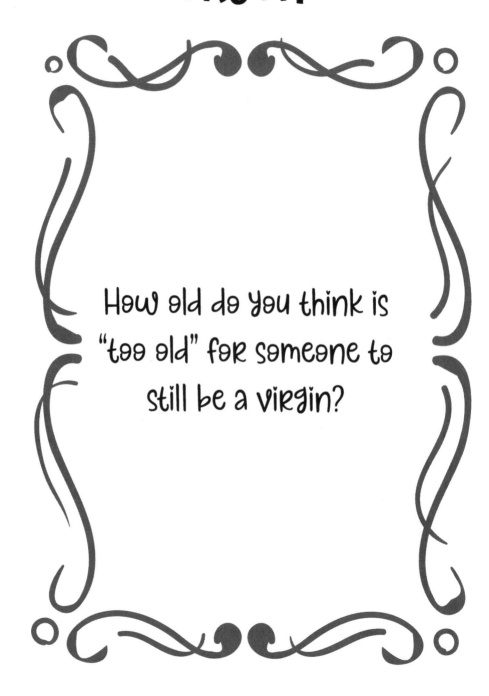

How old do you think is "too old" for someone to still be a virgin?

#20
DARE

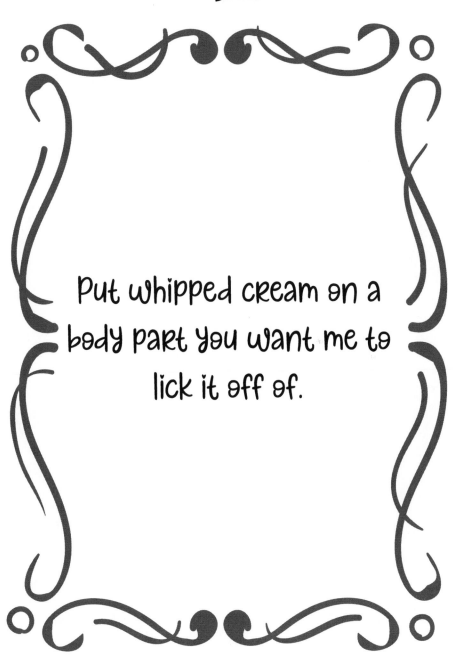

Put whipped cream on a
body part you want me to
lick it off of.

21
TRUTH

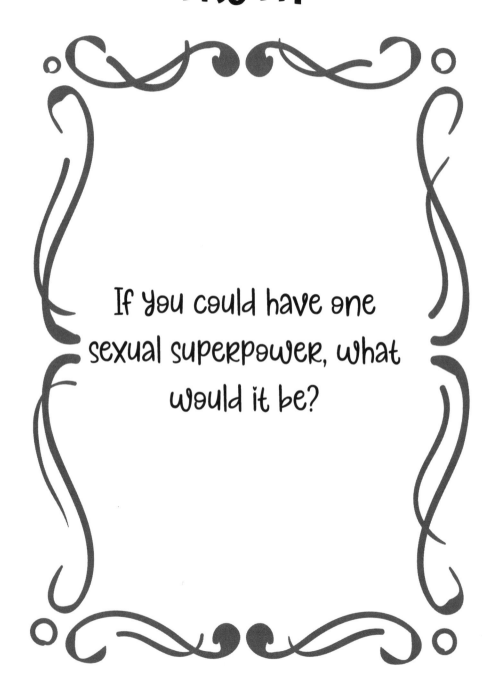

If you could have one
sexual superpower, what
would it be?

21
DARE

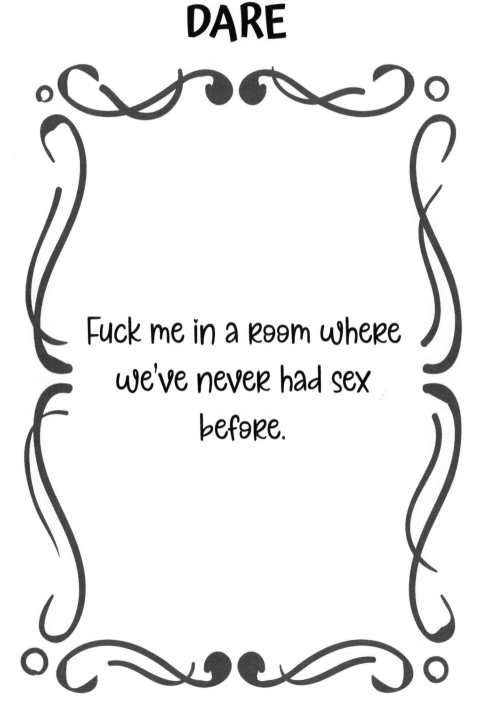

Fuck me in a room where
we've never had sex
before.

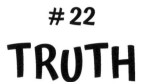

#22
TRUTH

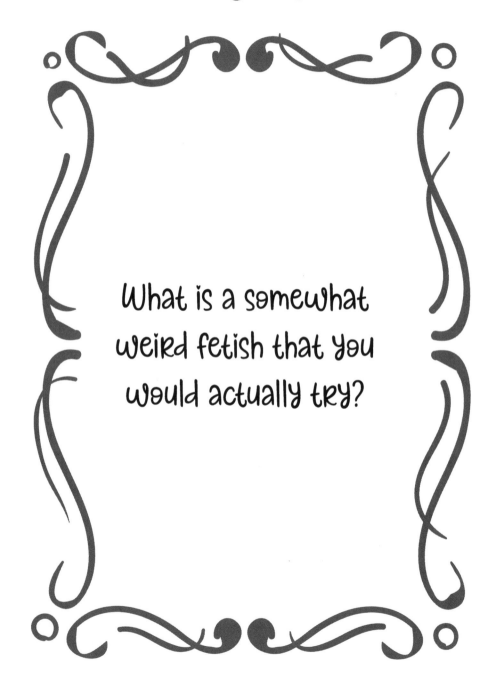

What is a somewhat weird fetish that you would actually try?

#22
DARE

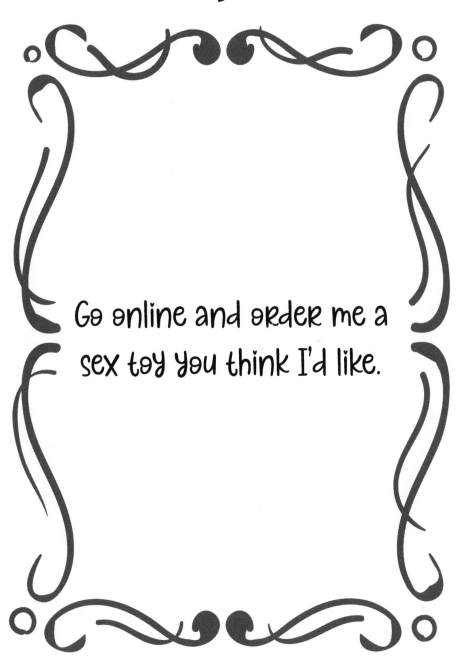

Go online and order me a
sex toy you think I'd like.

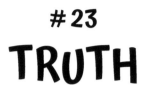

#23
TRUTH

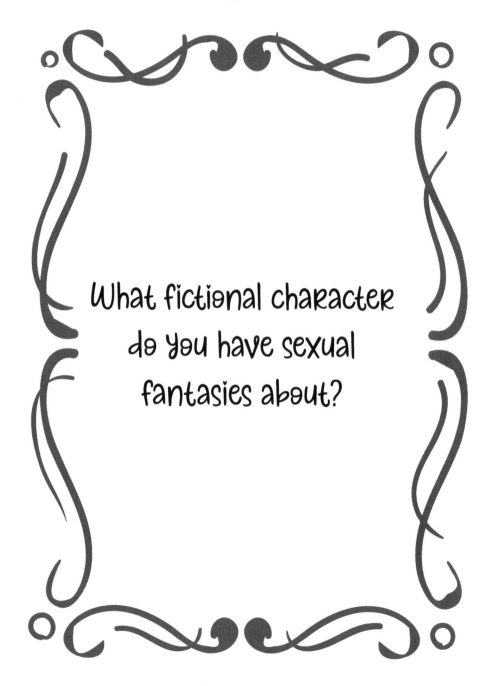

What fictional character
do you have sexual
fantasies about?

DARE

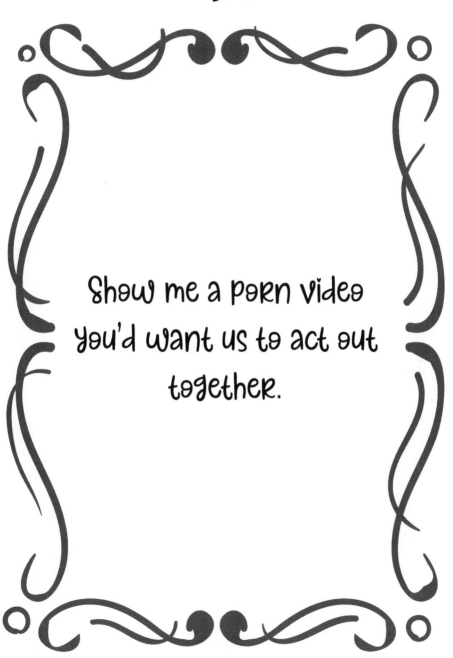

Show me a porn video
you'd want us to act out
together.

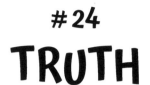

#24
TRUTH

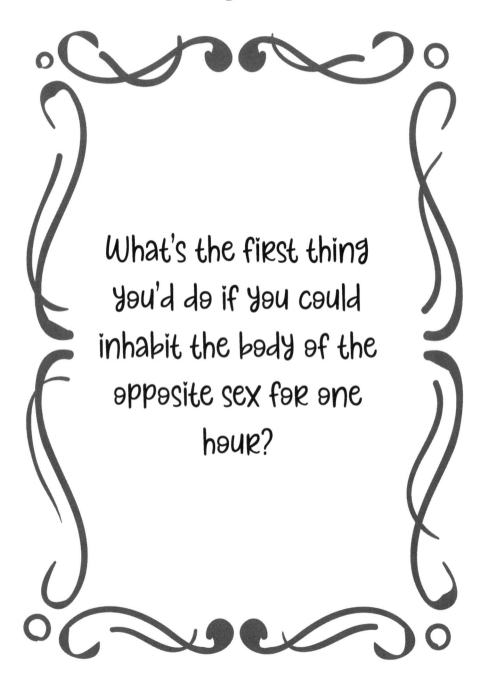

What's the first thing you'd do if you could inhabit the body of the opposite sex for one hour?

#24
DARE

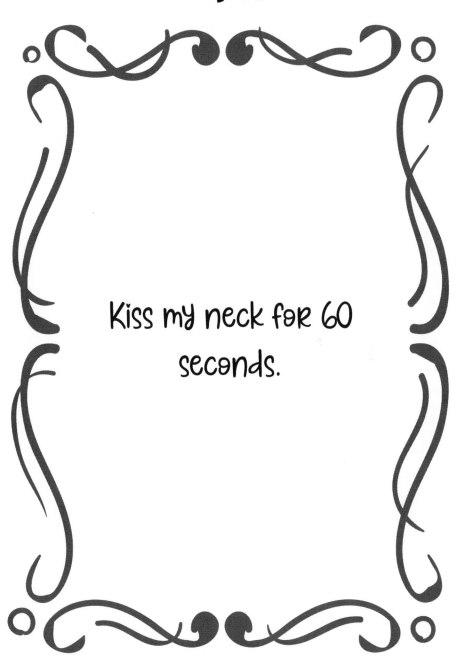

Kiss my neck for 60 seconds.

#25
TRUTH

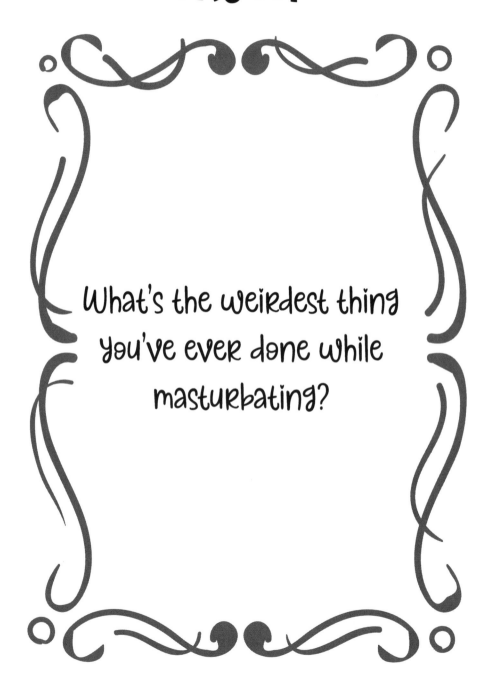

What's the weirdest thing
you've ever done while
masturbating?

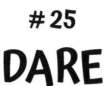

25
DARE

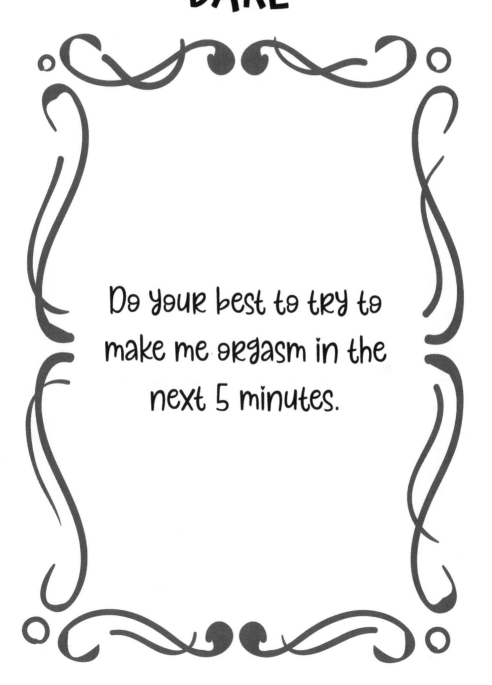

Do your best to try to make me orgasm in the next 5 minutes.

26
TRUTH

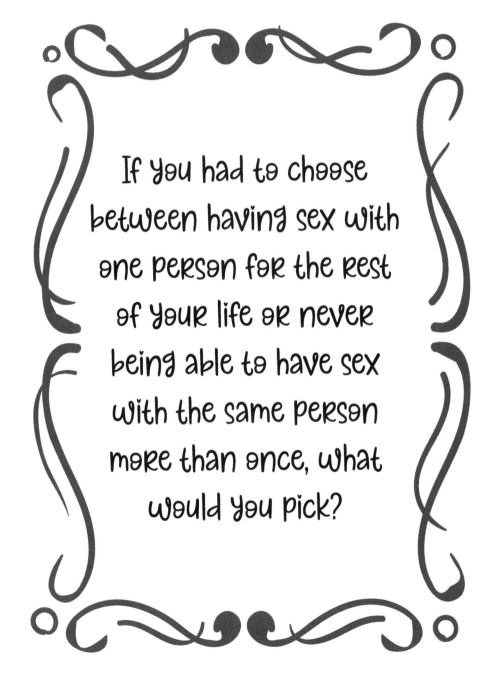

If you had to choose between having sex with one person for the rest of your life or never being able to have sex with the same person more than once, what would you pick?

26
DARE

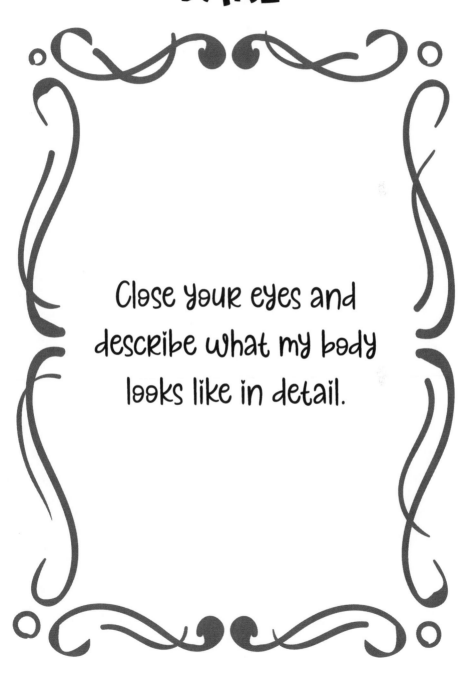

Close your eyes and
describe what my body
looks like in detail.

TRUTH

Would you rather pay someone to put on a striptease for you (they aren't allowed to touch), pay someone to cuddle and massage you while wearing non-sexy clothes, or pay someone to talk dirty over the phone but never be able to see them?

DARE

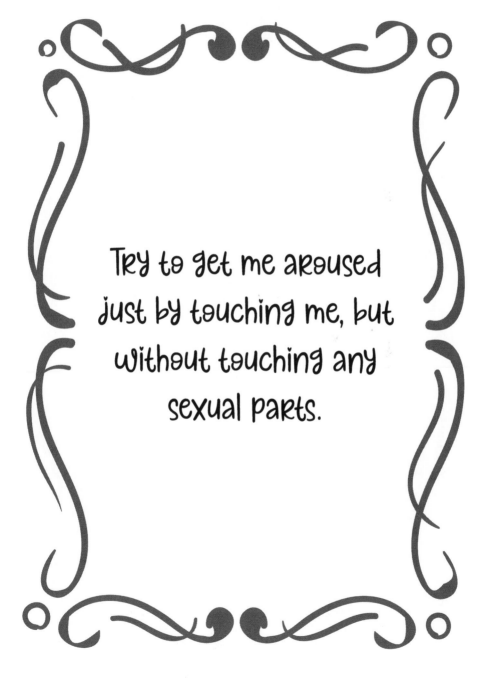

Try to get me aroused
just by touching me, but
without touching any
sexual parts.

TRUTH

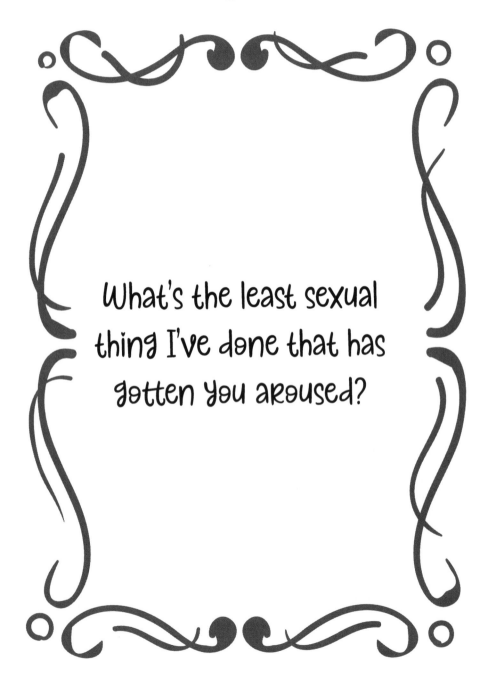

What's the least sexual thing I've done that has gotten you aroused?

28
DARE

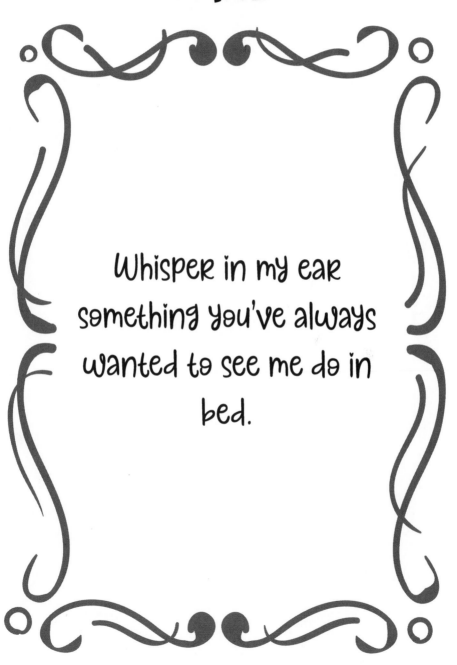

Whisper in my ear
something you've always
wanted to see me do in
bed.

TRUTH

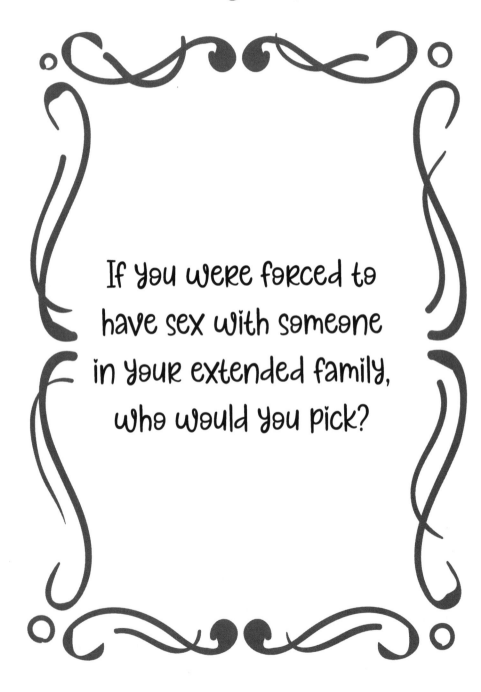

If you were forced to have sex with someone in your extended family, who would you pick?

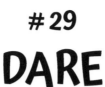

29
DARE

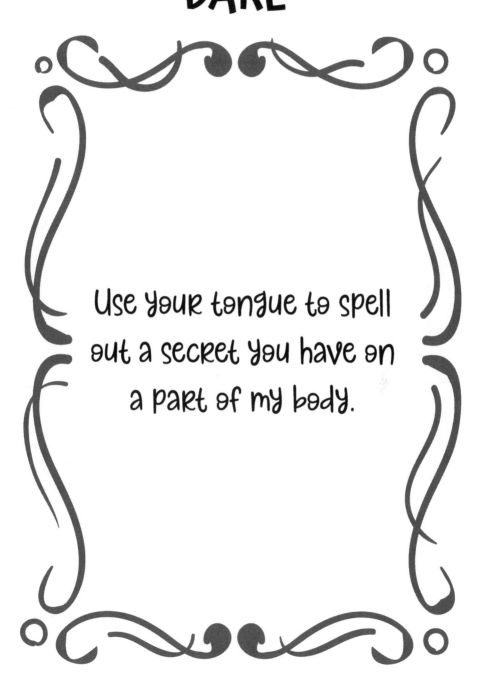

Use your tongue to spell
out a secret you have on
a part of my body.

#30
TRUTH

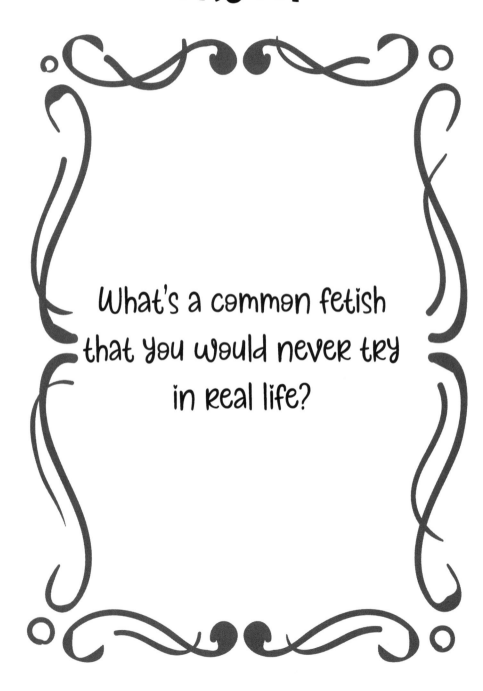

What's a common fetish
that you would never try
in real life?

#30
DARE

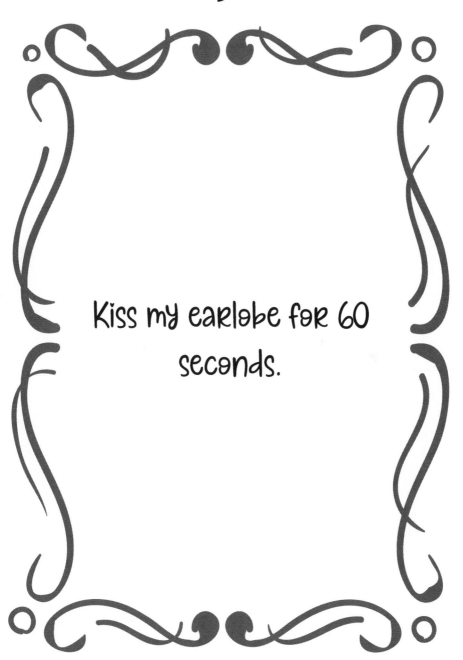

Kiss my earlobe for 60
seconds.

#31
TRUTH

What do you wish someone would have told you about sex way earlier?

DARE

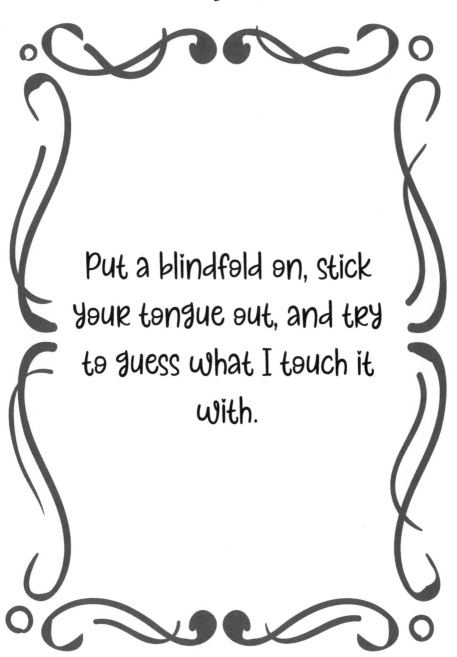

Put a blindfold on, stick your tongue out, and try to guess what I touch it with.

32

TRUTH

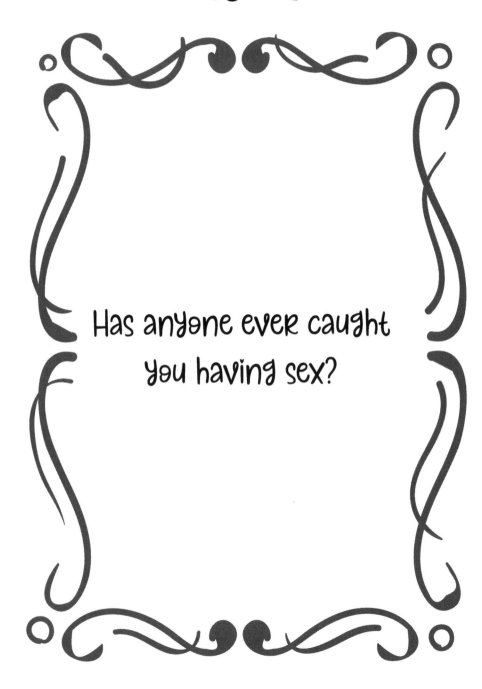

Has anyone ever caught
you having sex?

#32
DARE

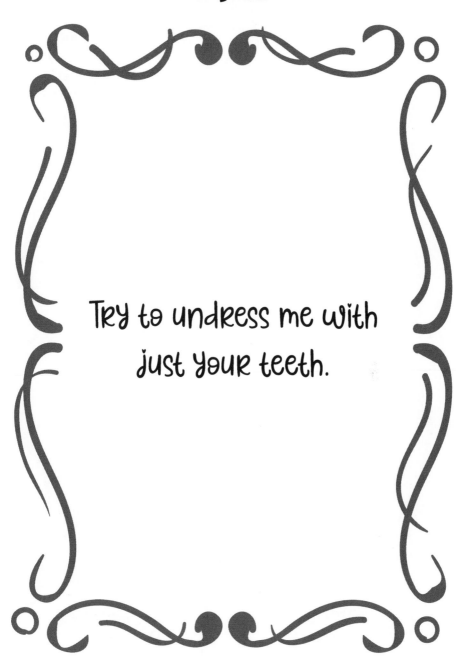

Try to undress me with just your teeth.

33
TRUTH

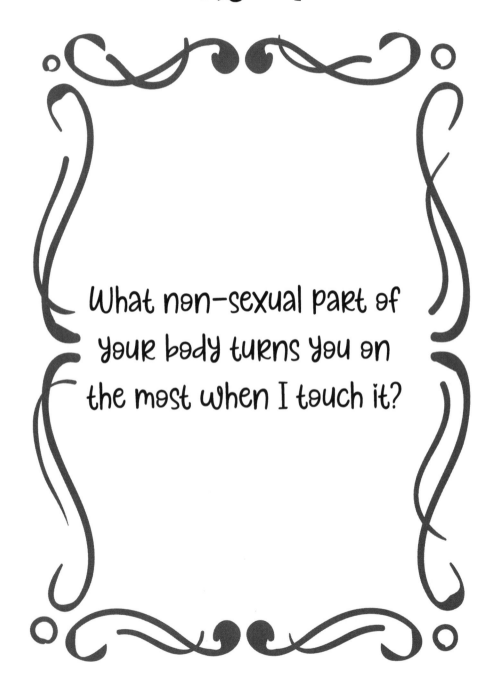

What non-sexual part of
your body turns you on
the most when I touch it?

#33
DARE

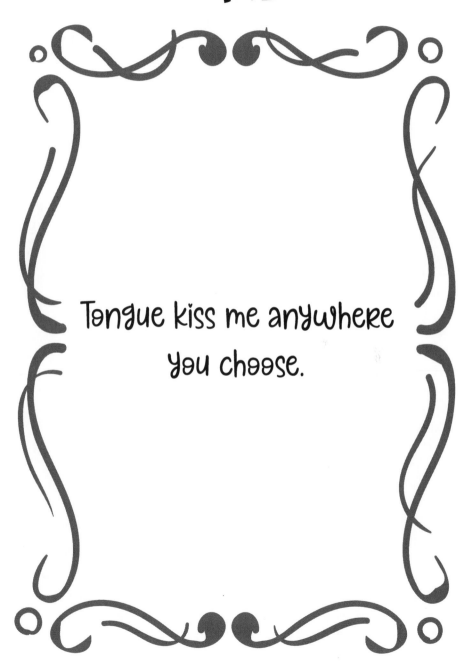

Tongue kiss me anywhere
you choose.

#34
TRUTH

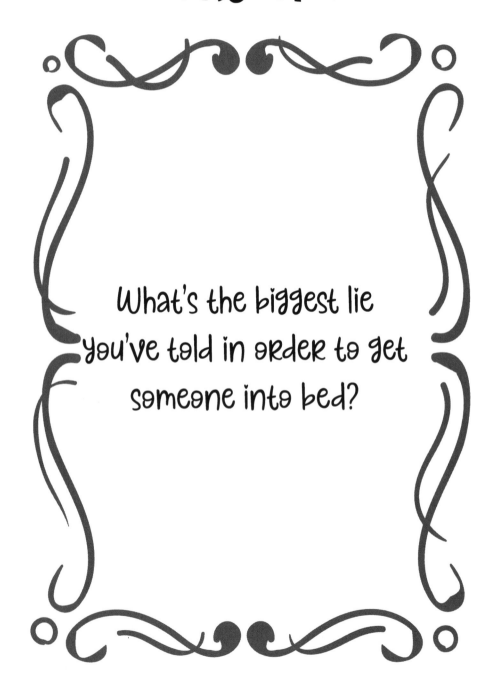

What's the biggest lie
you've told in order to get
someone into bed?

DARE

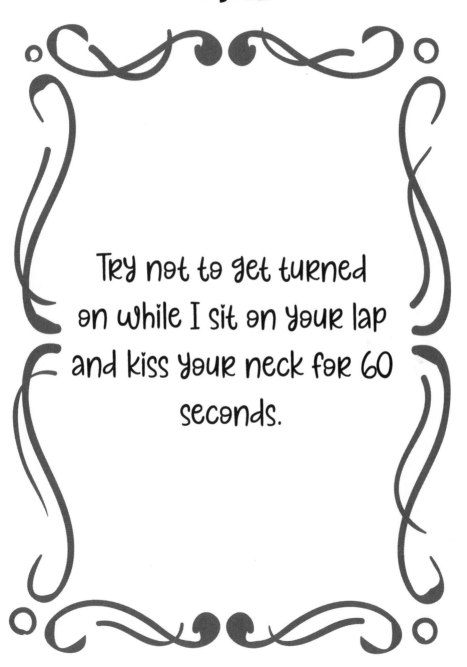

Try not to get turned on while I sit on your lap and kiss your neck for 60 seconds.

35
TRUTH

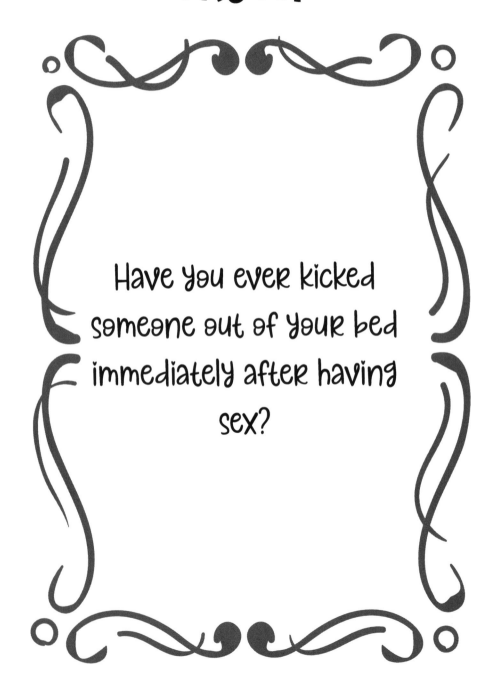

Have you ever kicked someone out of your bed immediately after having sex?

DARE

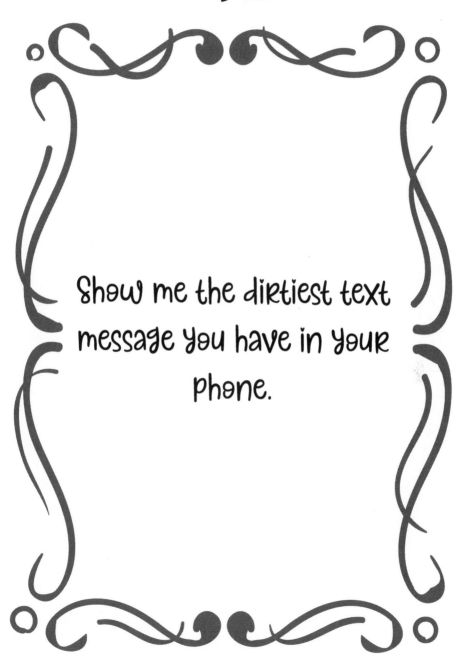

Show me the dirtiest text message you have in your phone.

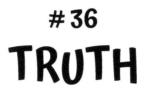

#36
TRUTH

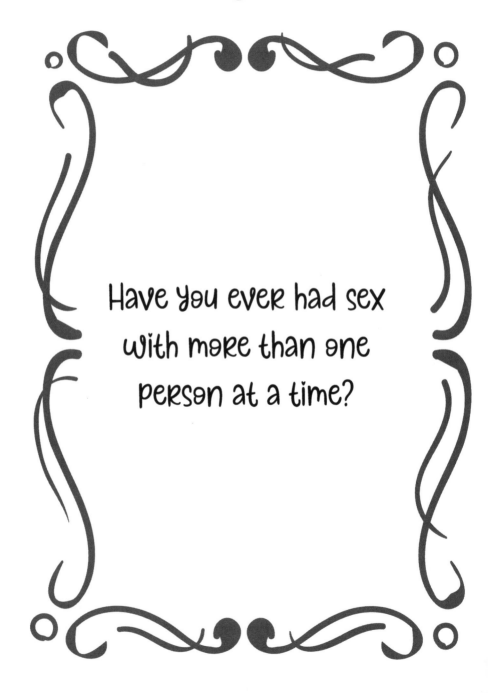

Have you ever had sex
with more than one
person at a time?

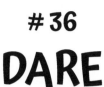

#36
DARE

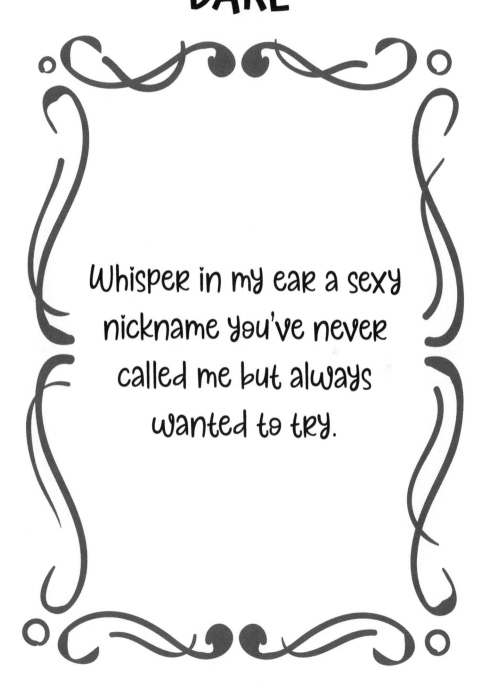

Whisper in my ear a sexy
nickname you've never
called me but always
wanted to try.

37
TRUTH

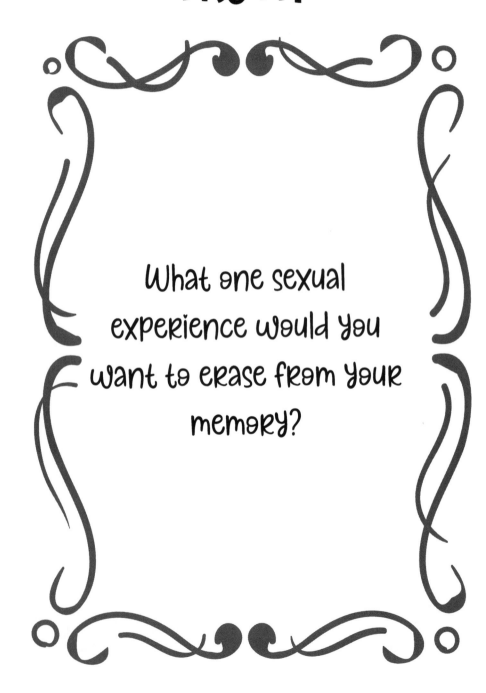

What one sexual experience would you want to erase from your memory?

#37
DARE

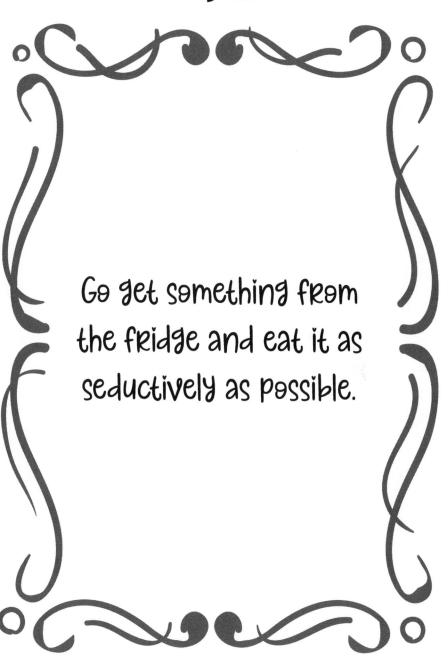

Go get something from
the fridge and eat it as
seductively as possible.

#38
TRUTH

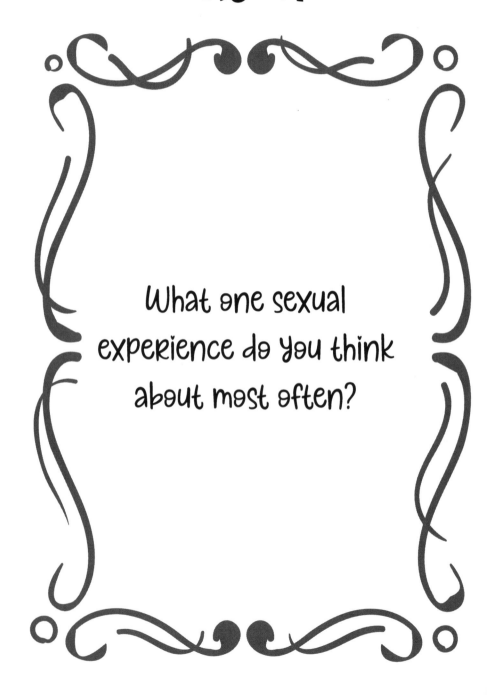

What one sexual
experience do you think
about most often?

DARE

For the rest of the game, pretend you are a cop who wants to arrest me for the crime of being too sexy.

39
TRUTH

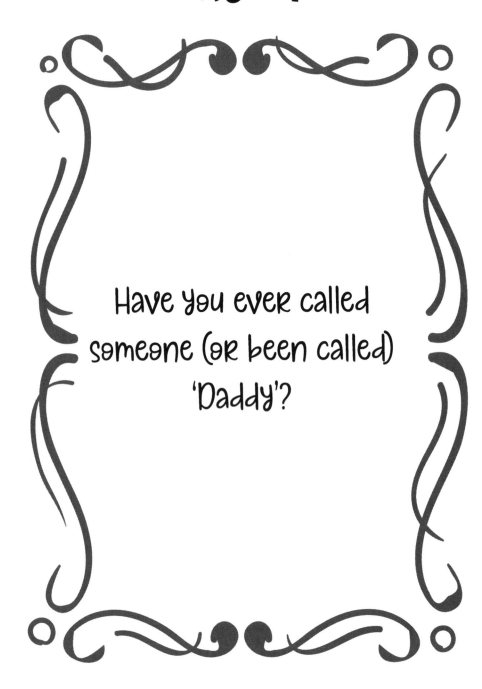

Have you ever called
someone (or been called)
'Daddy'?

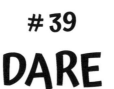

#39
DARE

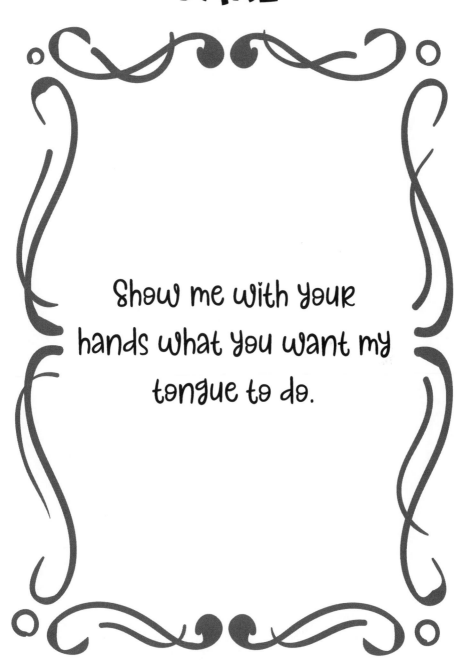

Show me with your
hands what you want my
tongue to do.

#40
TRUTH

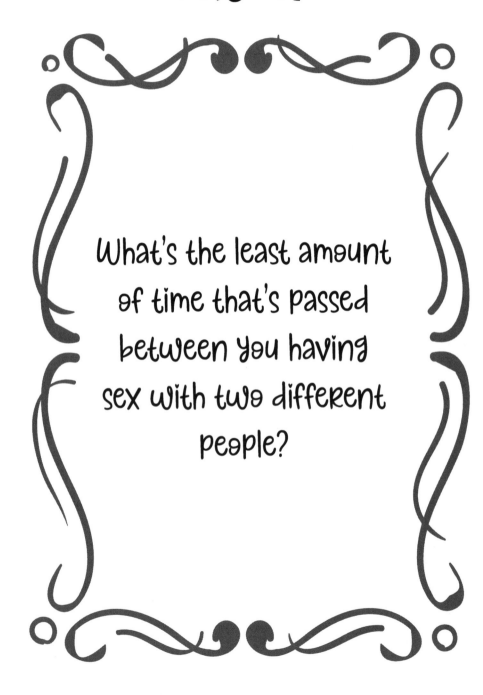

What's the least amount
of time that's passed
between you having
sex with two different
people?

#40
DARE

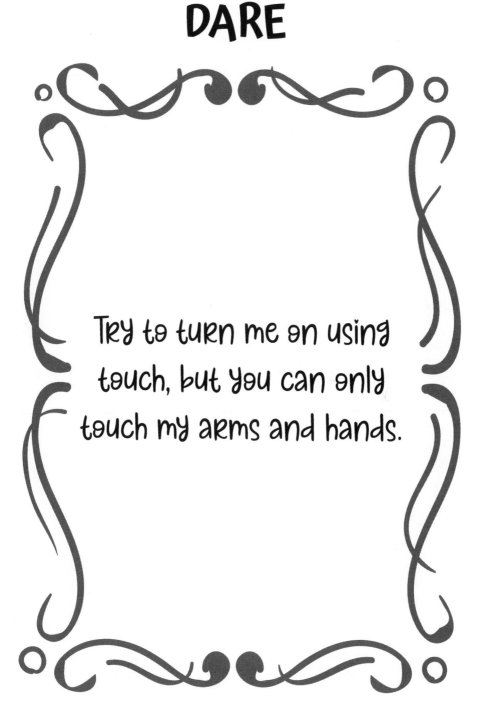

Try to turn me on using
touch, but you can only
touch my arms and hands.

41
TRUTH

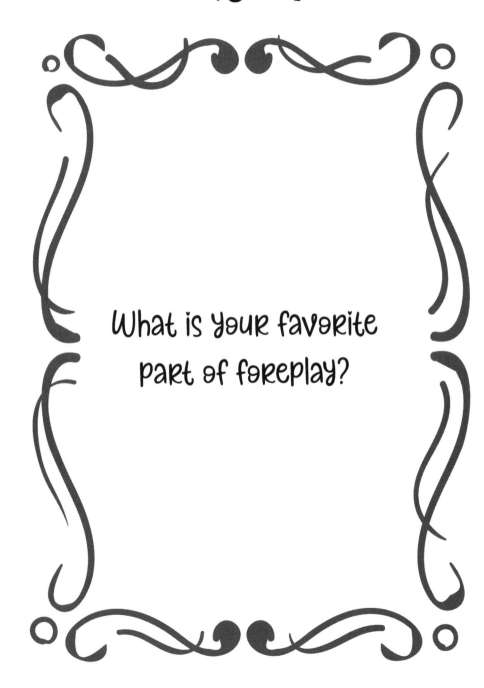

What is your favorite
part of foreplay?

41
DARE

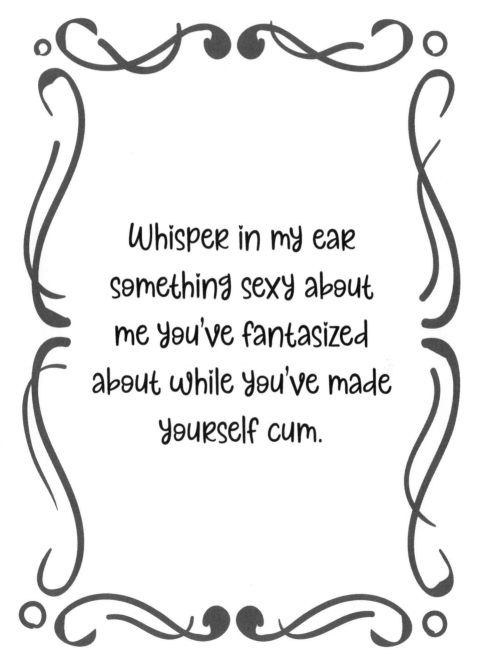

Whisper in my ear
something sexy about
me you've fantasized
about while you've made
yourself cum.

42
TRUTH

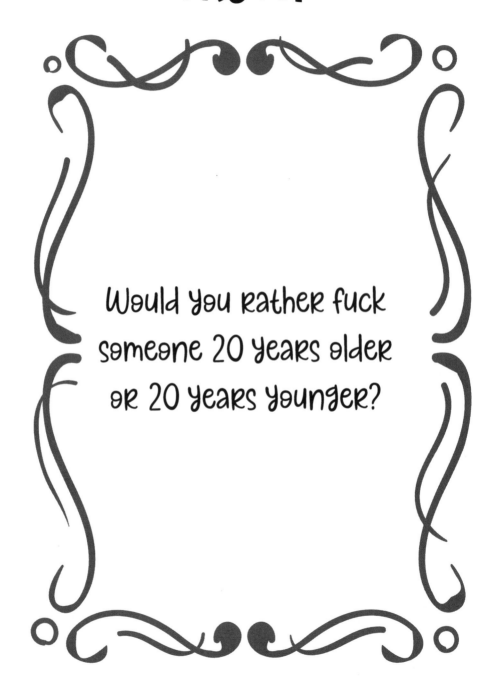

Would you rather fuck someone 20 years older or 20 years younger?

42
DARE

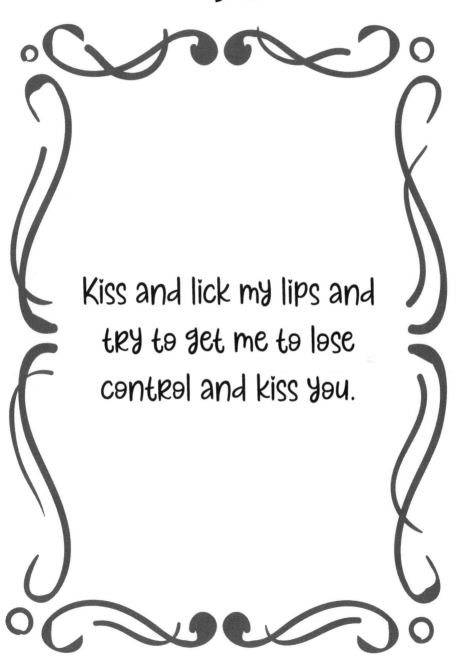

Kiss and lick my lips and try to get me to lose control and kiss you.

#43
TRUTH

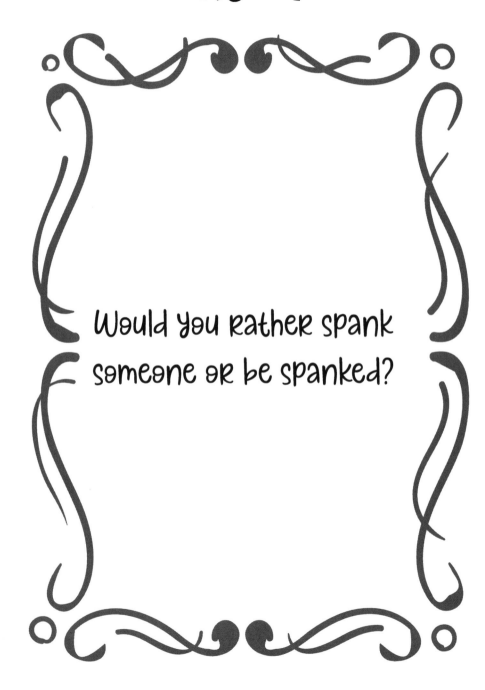

Would you rather spank someone or be spanked?

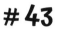

#43
DARE

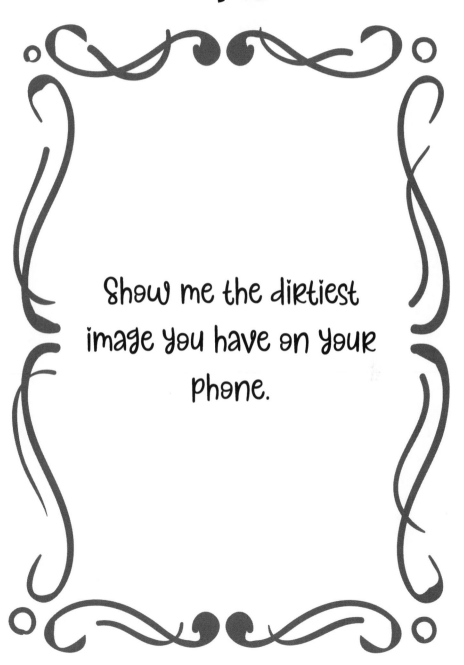

Show me the dirtiest
image you have on your
phone.

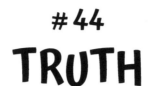

#44
TRUTH

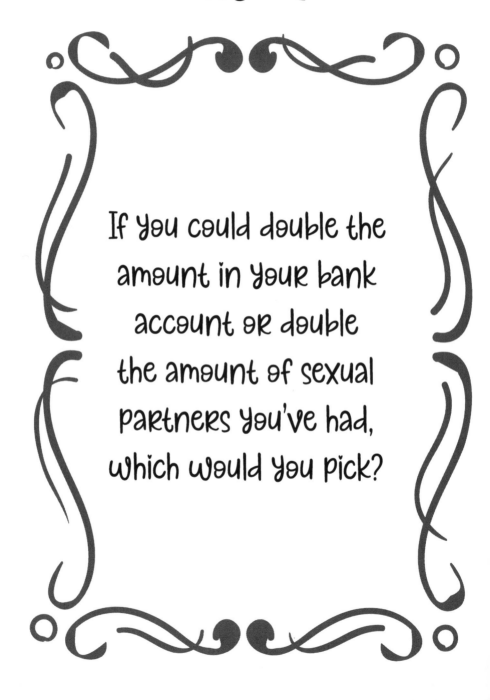

If you could double the amount in your bank account or double the amount of sexual partners you've had, which would you pick?

#44
DARE

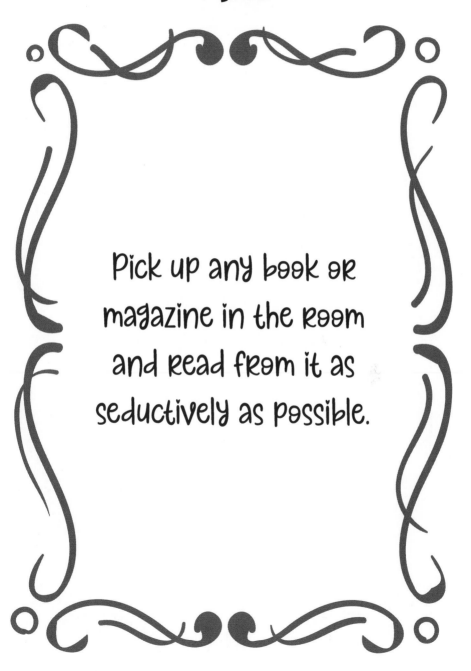

Pick up any book or
magazine in the room
and read from it as
seductively as possible.

TRUTH

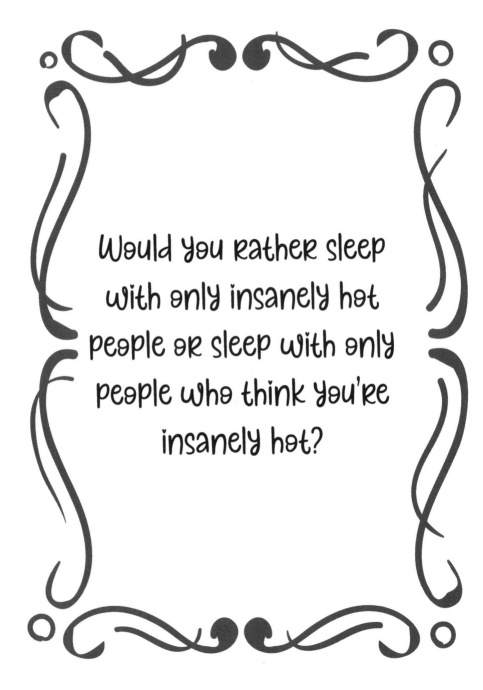

Would you rather sleep
with only insanely hot
people or sleep with only
people who think you're
insanely hot?

#45
DARE

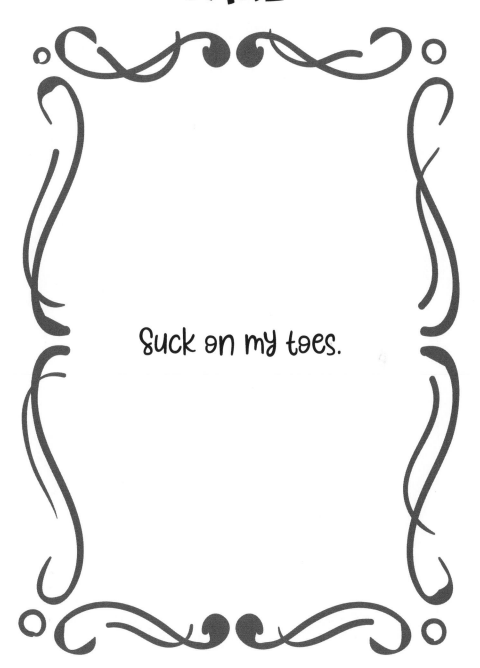

Suck on my toes.

46
TRUTH

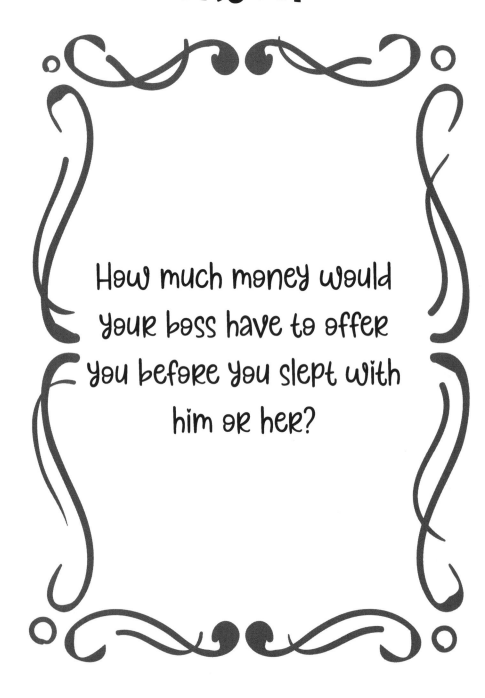

How much money would your boss have to offer you before you slept with him or her?

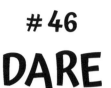

#46
DARE

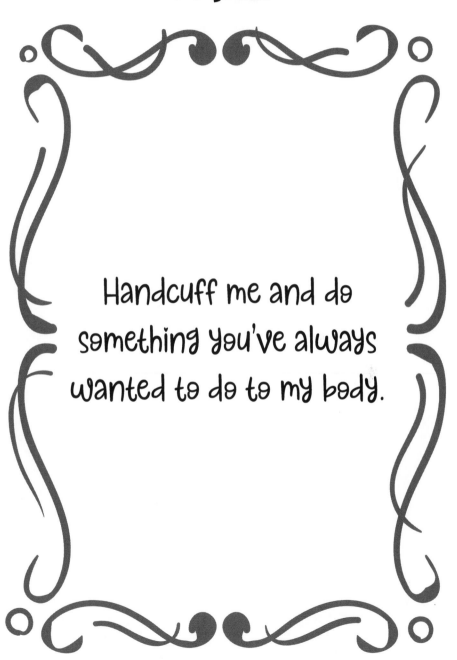

Handcuff me and do
something you've always
wanted to do to my body.

#47
TRUTH

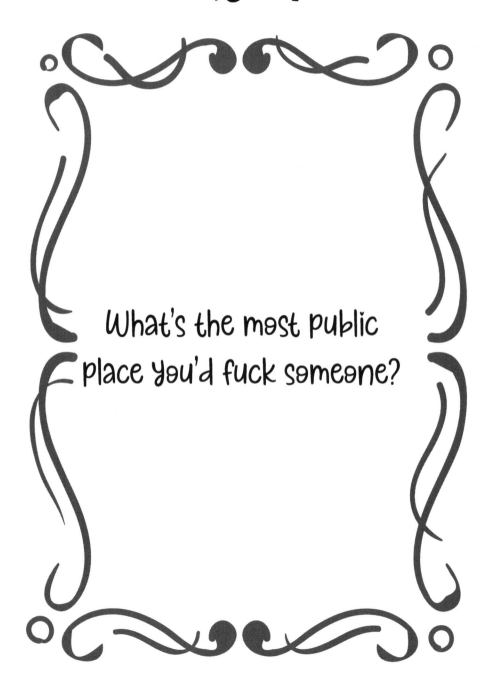

What's the most public place you'd fuck someone?

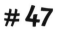

#47
DARE

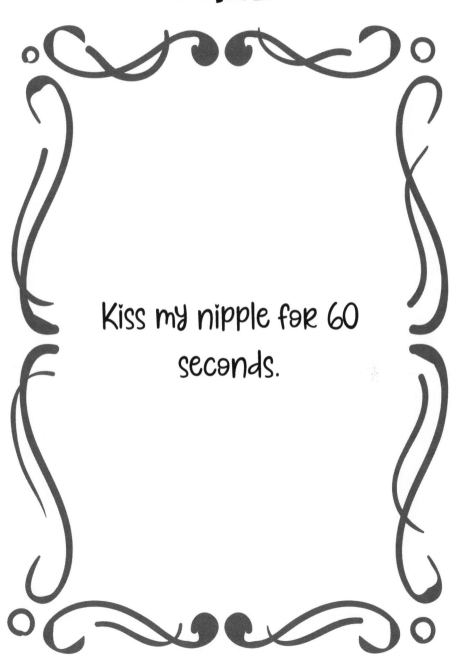

Kiss my nipple for 60
seconds.

#48
TRUTH

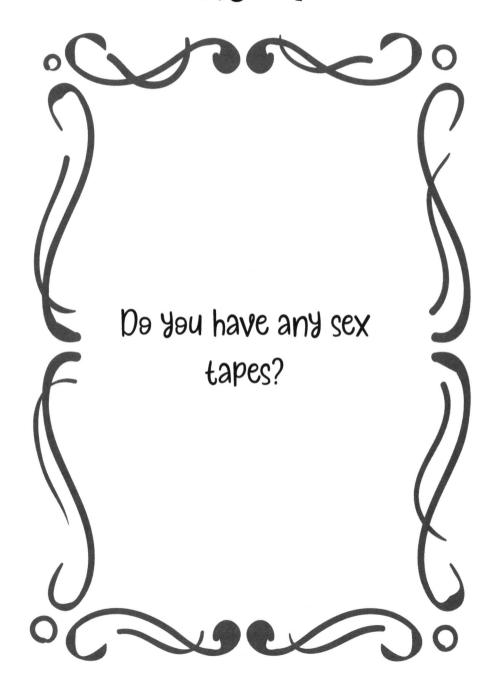

Do you have any sex
tapes?

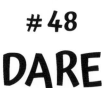

#48
DARE

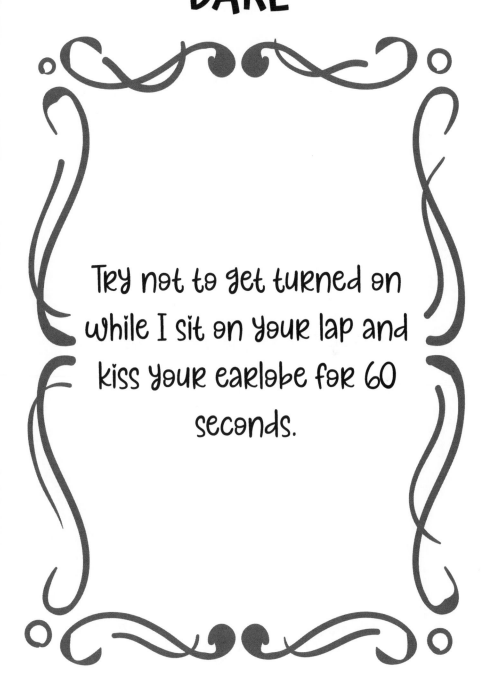

Try not to get turned on while I sit on your lap and kiss your earlobe for 60 seconds.

49
TRUTH

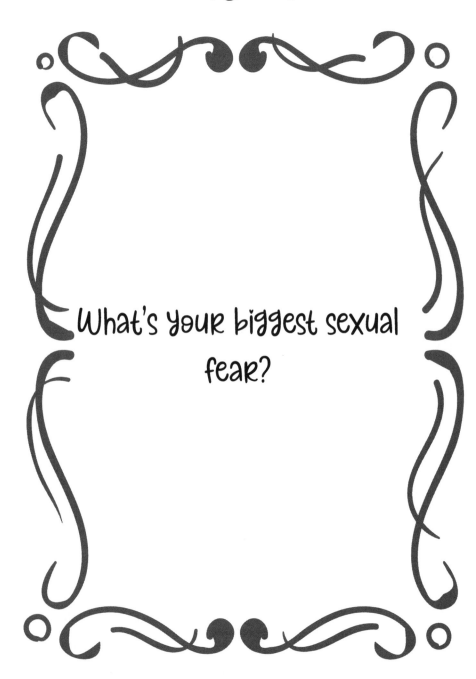

What's your biggest sexual fear?

#49
DARE

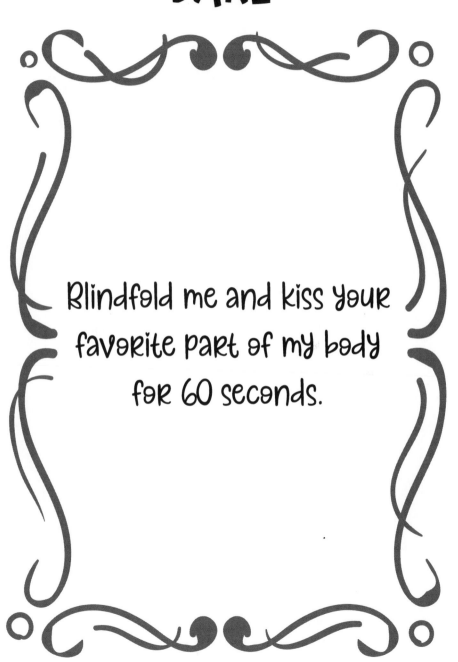

Blindfold me and kiss your
favorite part of my body
for 60 seconds.

#50
TRUTH

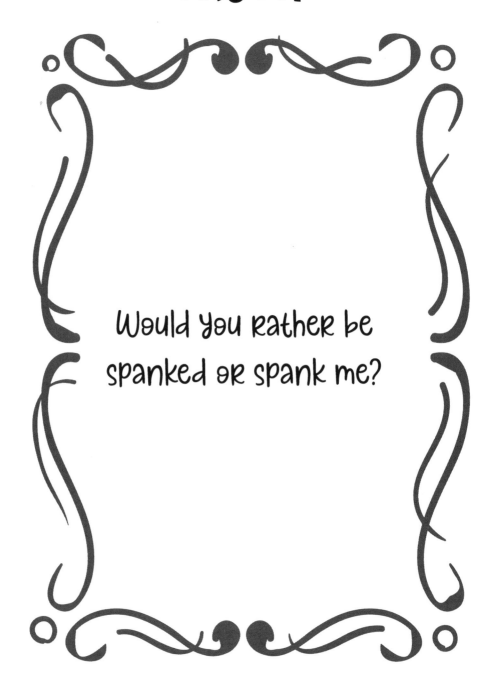

Would you rather be
spanked or spank me?

#50
DARE

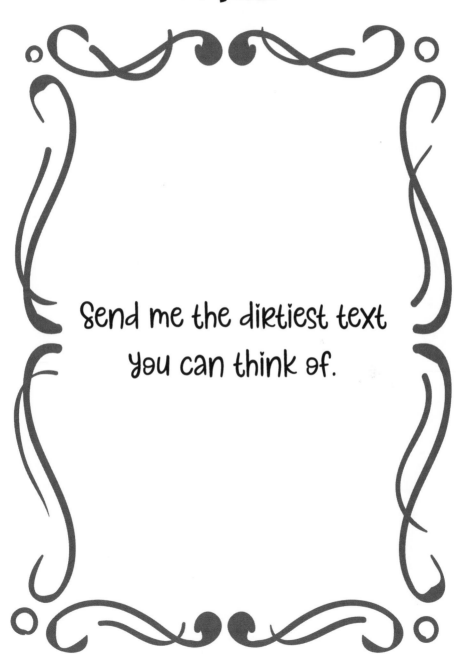

Send me the dirtiest text
you can think of.

Printed in Great Britain
by Amazon

14153001R00059